The International Behavioural and Social Sciences Library

THREE ESSAYS ON THE
PAINTING OF OUR TIME

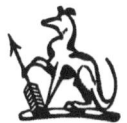

TAVISTOCK

PSYCHOLOGY OF ART: SELECTED WORKS OF ADRIAN STOKES
In 6 Volumes

THREE ESSAYS ON THE PAINTING OF OUR TIME

ADRIAN STOKES

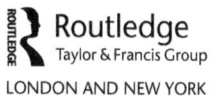 Routledge
Taylor & Francis Group

LONDON AND NEW YORK

First published in 1961 by
Tavistock Publications (1959) Limited

Reprinted in 2001 by
Routledge
2 Park Square, Milton Park, Abingdon, Oxon, OX14 4RN
711 Third Avenue, New York, NY 10017

Transferred to Digital Printing 2007

Routledge is an imprint of the Taylor & Francis Group

First issued in paperback 2013

British Library Cataloguing in Publication Data
A CIP catalogue record for this book
is available from the British Library

Three Essays on the Painting of our Time
ISBN13: 978-0-415-26494-5 (hardback)
ISBN13: 978-0-415-86601-9 (paperback)

Psychology of Art: Selected Works of Adrian Stokes: 6 Volumes
ISBN 0-415-26516-9
The International Behavioural and Social Sciences Library
112 Volumes
ISBN 0-415-25670-4

ADRIAN STOKES

Three
Essays
on the Painting
of our Time

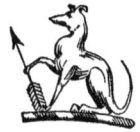

TAVISTOCK PUBLICATIONS

First published in 1961
by Tavistock Publications (1959) Limited
2 Park Square, Milton Park,
Abingdon, Oxon, OX14 4RN
in 11pt. Times Roman
by The Alcuin Press
Welwyn Garden City, Herts.

Acknowledgments

Thanks are due to Chatto and Windus for permission to quote from *The Doors of Perception* and *Heaven and Hell*, both by Aldous Huxley; to Thames and Hudson in respect of *The Concise History of Modern Painting*, by Herbert Read; and to the Editor of the *International Journal of Psycho-Analysis* in respect of papers by Hanna Segal and Elliott Jaques.

Contents

I. THE LUXURY AND NECESSITY OF PAINTING

I. The Luxury and Necessity of Painting

Not even those who detest art will be averse to the presence of picture galleries near luxurious shops. For a moment luxury may satisfy greed and provide the riches that separate us from loneliness. We sniff a bountiful air at shop windows, contemplating possessions not yet allotted, and sometimes unenviously any magnificence, the width of a street or the span of a doorway. Entertainment seeks to bring in train such bounty, experiences that are of the nature of meals; though they but symbolize suppers, surfeit supervenes. It comes about, then, that when we are at table we may hope to incorporate far more than our food; as we watch others they appear to reabsorb what we imagine to be predominant experiences. I have had this fantasy when watching directors of galleries that exhibit paintings, at a restaurant. It seemed that theirs was very fine nourishment, with associations that differed greatly from a stuffing or emparcelling: indeed, so enduring and so various is the luxurious stain upon directors of good paintings that their actual nourishment appears to lend them the overtones of lasting reassurance that may visit others only occasionally, should the satisfaction of various appetites coalesce in the pleasure of the table.

Of course good paintings are extremely valuable, a richness that lends itself to these imaginative richnesses. The gallery director has them on his walls. He may suffer from various difficulties in connection with food; nevertheless, a modicum of the fantasy of the luxuriousness of his eating will, I am sure, occasionally at least, be his as well.

To his sanctum I attribute some Italian Baroque paintings,

1

small, boldly painted with the raw touches that will eventually prove to have heralded the modern pictorial era. The canvases were studies and sketches for large paintings, or for their details. In one a mushroom cloud of angels grows, as it were from the compost of an ecstatic saint who grovels upward from below: the picture vibrates with rays of a sudden flowering, but lines in one corner indicate a hard architecture, the pillars and the underside of a cornice whose grooved, stepped mass embraces the shrinking or resurgence of figures as does a basin that both holds and spills the fountain's play. The union is ennobling, an interchange or commerce we would have in ourselves between passions and the stone, since the architecture symbolizes our rational disposition unberated by death and decay, embodies a Parnassus-like bent whereby proportion and space envelop our emotions, dispersing litter on a desk and the rhythmless rush of noises from the street that link us to a chaos, otherwise inescapable, throughout the length and breadth of London ever ignoble where this painting is noble.How few are the colonnades, those tunnels with pierced sides, how small the perpetuity of silent flank and orifice, how little by which to recognize our own ideal states. . . . As well as of the rational disposition, a good building is the monument to physique.

But it is unlikely that this director has much interest in architecture: it is not necessary today for devotees of painting: they do not acknowledge building to be the root of any grandeur and the presiding genius of graphic art. The lapse is due to failure, and to a resurgence that is taut, of architecture in our time; even more because, in view of this failure from the middle of the last century, painting, while avoiding as a rule an obvious architectural balance, has itself been inspired to fill the void, to provide the more intimate architectural pleasures, striving to envelop and to feed us without ceremony by means of clamant textures, to enwrap us with a surface, to drive us by shock into a place of safety, to declaim

2

from a wall the need for tactile passages and transitions that
were once available in lovely streets. The primacy of architecture, mother of the arts, is not first as the school of proportion and design but as the universal witness to the luxuries
of art, to the aesthetic translation of mental process, as well
as the scenes of living, into the terms of an absorbable substance, or of our envelopment by an object. But simultaneously there exists an emphasis upon the separateness of the
artifact, upon the cake that survives our eating of it. Thus, in
the name of object self-sufficiency and corporeal wholeness,
art may bestow another luxury in the enshrinement of even
the greatest misery, a luxury gained from the putting together
of fragments of experience that have been dispersed, so that
even pain coheres, owns features: a service is done thereby, a
good restored. Graphic boldness and idiosyncrasy satisfy
more people today than fine building surrounded by ill-
advised curves and strong material and dreary roofs and the
blatant, negative pretension of all urban scenes. Surely there
has never before been so sterling and durable a debasement,
multiplied in instances by the million, of members and
materials that were once well used. It will be some time before
late Victorian and Edwardian miasmas will have yielded their
present air of universality.

Envelopment by building, by street, is almost unknown to
Englishmen as a reassurance, but is universal in experiences
of confusion or of the drugs that alleviate, such as the droplet
comfort in a cottage roof, in a quaint lamp-post or a causeway
too windswept for advertisements. Even so, our director has
enjoyed visits to Rome; his pleasure in his Baroque paintings
reminds him of cobbled roads and their smooth houses with
apertures that are tall: and he has read in Wittkower of a
conscious Baroque aim to envelop the spectator. 'With
Caravaggio the great gesture had another distinct meaning;
it was a psychological device, not unknown in the history of
art, to draw the beholder into the orbit of the picture . . .

3

Bernini's St. Theresa, shown in rapture, seems to be sus-
pended in mid-air, and this can only appear as reality by
virtue of the implied visionary state of mind of the beholder
. . . Miracles, wondrous events, supra-natural phenomena are
given an air of verisimilitude' (Wittkower, 1958). The power
of this art to envelop us suggests confidence in the phantasy
that an interchange infuses the complexity of relationship
between substances themselves, between objects, between
different arts though employed to represent a single vivid
happening. Architecture, sculpture, painting merge in the
representation of St. Theresa's ecstasy, just as river-god, shell,
dolphin are as one with the water of the Barberini fountain.

Architecture is limited to forms without events; in many
styles or periods an architectural exemplar has provided the
model for translating graphic subjects into the terms of a
concatenation built upon a ground bass. There are Italian
masterpieces, for instance the operas of Vincenzo Bellini,
whose continuous simplicity remains poignant, whose lyric-
ism remains unmatched in a firmness far from romantic, sug-
gesting sunlit or shaded loggias and above them, upon the
wall, smooth apertures that give light, and above again the
jutting features of a cornice-head.

The churches of Rome reign easily over the noisiest traffic
in the world; even in this wretched sanctum in the West End
of London, the Baroque paintings lend a Theatine quiet un-
separated from the life of the town, as if a burst pipe that
floods a building's face in patches might yet convey the image
of a spring. We hang our paintings to convert not only our
houses but our neighbourhoods and our neighbours.

Little understood by our director, the Baroque paintings
are a side-line relegated to this narrow room. Modern paintings are his livelihood and his life. Let us go into the galleries.
There he is, in the hour before the midday meal, doubtless
still stimulated by pictures whose appeal fails only at the tap
of another example. They titillate the appetite to absorb all

4

things: who can say where limitation lies since these artists' aims have been to show the unknown as uniform in strong impact with the known? We have here the manner of endless bodily function as well as of hardly touched states of mind, more muscular, more independent than the resonance of images in a dream yet, when viewed in terms of the intellect's categories, vague and boundless as are the spongy images of sleep so often tied to an inconsequent context, equalled occasionally by the name the modern artist puts upon his painting in the catalogue.

'I no longer invite the spectator to walk into my canvases,' writes the American Action painter, Grace Hartigan (1959), 'I want a surface that resists, like a wall, not opens like a gate'. The wall, Leonardo's homogeneous wall with adventitious marks which, he said, encourage fantasy to reinforce their suggestion, has been an especial spur from the time of the Impressionists, from the time of the new negative significance of buildings in our epoch for which the picture plane, the picture surface, has become an affirmative substitute; so much is this so that much modern painting ceases to have parts or pieces, in the sense of parts that when abstracted from the whole would remain objects of beauty as of value. What price a section of an Action painting (of one section rather than another), or even of a Cubist painting or a Mondrian? The modern stress upon unity and purity, upon strict aesthetic relevance, connotes a stress upon homogeneity: in some styles the picture plane in fact resembles a blank wall to which is entrusted the coalescence of dissonances or blows directed at the spectator. Even when this is not so, we are likely to discover the kindred notion of something unlimited. Unspoken experiences, bodily and mental, have always been incorporated into art through the appeal of formal relationships: but when, as now, they are offered without the accompaniment of any other symbolic content—or if there is another programme, when it is distorted or simplified even

5

to a greater extent than in a style that has been strictly conventionalized—they readily suggest the unlimited, a concept always present to the mind in terms of a boundless, traumatic bad or a boundless, bountiful good, by which we suffer envelopment or from which we would perpetually feed.

Now, the simplest relationships, the most sporadic marks, have deep meaning: we have been shown it beyond all question. We have today an art without manners, without veneer, arresting, knock-you-down yet unbraced and unlimited, it appears, in scope: that is one reason why it must continually change so much: what is novel affords a sense of boundless possibility with which we may exchange ourselves in lieu of achievement. Modern art tends thus to be romantic, somewhat at the expense of the other fundamental draw of the work of art, as a self-sufficient entity, though this character too has been isolated and worked upon. The palpable textures of modern painting express the division and disintegration of culture as well as the ambivalent artist's restitution, often carried no further than an assembly of scaffolding. We are then left with an unceremonious image that seems to symbolize the process of art itself, of the hidden content, always immanent, whereby mere space and shape touch in us sensations of pain, struggle, anxiety, or joy that we have already begun to translate into tactile and even visual sensations, since a parallel amalgam is ceaselessly registered in some part of the mind. Appreciation is a mode of recognition: we recognize but we cannot name, we cannot recall by an effort of will: the contents that reach us in the terms of aesthetic form have the 'feel' of a dream that is otherwise forgotten. This 'feel' too may be lost until it is recalled by an action in the street, by some concatenation of movement or of substances: in just this way much modern art offers us the 'feel' of our own structure, sometimes overriding the communication of particular feelings. Painting usually presents as well a specific subject-matter equivalent to the manifest content of a dream, in terms of an image of the waking world. The painter has been happiest when surrounded by an actual architecture which provided an assumption (a living style) that made it unnecessary to reconstruct *ab initio* for every work the rudiments of the body and of the psyche. Titian was adorning, not creating, the stone Venice, and Rembrandt the new Amsterdam. Architecture in the West has been the prime embodiment not only of art but of culture. There are left, of course, many beautiful places, many ordinary houses that are satisfying, particularly in the South; but it is not our ruling culture that creates them. Marinetti considered all the beauty of Italy an obstacle to his harsh idealization of the machine by which alone he felt enveloped in the unlimited way he demanded.

We will agree that the work of art is a construction. Inasmuch as man both physically and psychologically is a structure carefully amassed, a coalescence and a pattern, a balance imposed upon opposite drives, building is likely to be not only the most common but the most general symbol of our living and breathing: the house, besides, is the home and the symbol of the Mother: it is our upright bodies built cell by cell: a ledge is the foot, the knee and the brow. While we project our own being on to all things, the works of man, particularly houses or any of the shelters he inhabits, reflect ourselves more directly than will inorganic material that has not been cultivated thus. Of course buildings and the engineering involved, roads, bridges, and the rest, are so common as to be a part of a ceaseless environment. The ordered stone or brick encloses and defines: whether we will it or not, the eye explores these surfaces as if compelled to consult an oracle, the oracle of spatial relationships and of the texture that they serve. Hurt, hindered, and inspired by wall and ledge, the graphic artist has bestowed upon flat surfaces an expressiveness of space, volume, and texture equivalent to the impact, at the very least, of phantasies, events, moods. Architecture has provided the original terms of this 'language' that can rarely be put into words, though words may some-times be found for the simple employment of the 'language' by building when taken in conjunction with the natural scene. For instance, in the fascination of gazing along a dark passage into the outside light that invades an entrance, in a subject not uncommon for seventeenth-century Dutch painters, we may become aware that we contemplate under an image of dark, calm enclosure and of seeping light, the traumatic struggles that accompany our entry and our exit, in birth and death. To look along the walls of a cave into the blinding entry would be to experience a more dramatic symbol except for the consideration that a thousand threads of conscious life bring now to the passage and to the house, to the con-stricted brick or stone, an appropriate association. Seeing that the projection of phantasy on to all the phenomena of Nature is ceaseless, I would not deny that the 'language' of form must have a far wider origin; but I would claim that the example of building, not least in view of a context in the natural scene, has greatly served the precision of that 'language'; nor is it irrelevant that the graphic arts have been expended in many cultures on the adornment of building; nor that in pictorial art there has often figured the architectural organization. In almost all periods and styles buildings have been represented in painting: this is due not only to their commonness or to relevance for many scenes: a study of the employment of the architectural background in Renaissance art and in the theatre, shows without question that they are treated as the emblems both of ordered beauty and of a psychological tenor, in general as the presiding example of the conversion of phantasy into substance and for bestowing upon phantasy an autonomous and enduring body.

I shall now leave the terms of architecture and of luxury and our gallery director who loves luxury, achieves it from painting while more or less blind to building. I take leave of him because of the great distance between gallery and studio,

8

between art as luxury and art as necessity, though the former meaning is dependent upon, and founded upon, the latter.

The calm, the architecture, the luxury of pictures, what are they to the artist? Everything, I dare to say, though the making of art is a compulsive fruit of conflict, grief, and loss, of a sadness or a lack too old and bitter, too keen though hidden, to carry for long any romantic overtone. These feelings, the spring of art whatever an artist's overt temperament may be, correspond with our own feelings of loss and confusion: none of us has escaped them; hence the reassurance and luxury, since a synthesis and restitution will have been forged in the studio.

I do not want to hint that the artist should paint with tears rolling down cheeks, misting vision, but that he projects with astuteness upon the canvas an inner need in terms of the outside objects he has chosen, so that both he and they renew life; that is, so as to figure forth a pattern wherein confusion, though it be rehearsed there, may not rule; and greed and sadistic control of the object, though they too may figure, are not unchallenged.

We have no difficulty in speaking of the painter as the artist *par excellence*, of painting as the representative of art in general. I think that this is because of the instrument, the brush, tipped with the creative material, and because the canvas is worked at arm's length, with the result that the very act of painting as well as the pre-occupation with the representation of space, symbolize not only the restitutive process but a settled distance of the ego from its objects. The distance from us of our world varies continuously: the artist brings all into view, into focus, at arm's length as it were. Throughout consciousness one thing stands for another: we traffic all the time with symbols, in thought as well as in emotion; for, behind any feeling, behind the 'feel' of any argument even, there lurks another that is older and, as we proceed back, that is nearer to the source of its power over us. More than the rest of us, the artist is aware that what we see symbolizes the history as well as the aspiration of the mind: his task is to discover for them a felicitous embodiment in the outside world so that they be recognized as any object of perception is known, and better known the better the character of the object or scene represented has been seized in paint.

I am not necessarily referring to an artist's manifest aim but to the springs of his compulsion; nor do I refer in this context to anything that throws light on the immense variety of art, on the need for change. One of our most comprehensive symbolic objects—the artist is very aware of it—is the culture in which we live. In one aspect, culture and society are foods just as art itself is a food, an absorbable structure that nourishes our own. The artist absorbs his 'times', 'what is in the air'. On the other hand culture is recognized as an entity in the terms of the art it inspires; differences of culture are often measured succinctly in terms of art: and art itself, as a history of development and as a model of achievement, is another comprehensive object that the artist will tend to incorporate. Symbolic activities, art in chief, have their richest material in what is already richly and widely symbolic: the outermost ripple on the pond after the stone was cast is the one that most vividly reveals the power of the throwing and of the thing thrown. It seems that contemporary attitudes and achievements, whether or not we are sympathetic to them, provide indispensable terms for creativeness. It is well known that old works of art vary to some extent in their power of evocation, in accordance with their apparent comment upon a present cultural endeavour: and that the 'climate' of feeling is an inescapable framework for aesthetic emotion.

Our relationships to all objects seem to me to be describable in the terms of two extreme forms, the one a very strong identification with the object, whether projective or introjective, whereby a barrier between self and not-self is undone, the other a commerce with a self-sufficient and independent object at arm's length. In all times except the earliest weeks of life, both of these relationships, in vastly differing amalgams, are in play together, as is shown not only by psycho-analysis but by art, since the work of art is *par excellence* a self-sufficient object as well as a configuration that we absorb or to which we lend ourselves as manipulators. (The first generic difference between styles lies in the varying combinations by which these two extremes are conveyed to us). Here is to be observed a fundamental connection of art with the culture from which it arises; for, art helps us both to identify ourselves with some aspect of our culture, to incorporate cultural activities or to reject them, and at the same time to contemplate them as if they were fixed and hardy objects. From the angle of contemplation culture *is* art—hence, once more, the necessity of having art—since culture is most easily seen as an object for contemplation in aesthetic terms. Moreover, a cultural reconciliation of what is various, and even opposite, is perceived, when reflected in art, as a symbol for the integration that we have carried out upon contrary urges, opposite feelings, once widely separated, about one and the same person. In painting his picture the artist performs an act of integration upon the outside world that has reference, then, as well as to the independence of objects, first to the re-creation and to some resolution of his own inner processes, next in regard to the organization of the ego in a generalized sense, and finally in regard to a cultural significance. The result is an interplay between these modes of organization to the end of making one of them more poignant since it possesses the services of the others. Romantic art underlines an aspect of the artist's personality, Hellenic art the generous ideal of ego-integration, a severely conventionalized art, such as the Byzantine in a characteristic phase, the cultural hierarchy. Throughout the history of art, emphasis has more commonly lain here: art has been employed to mark ritual and religion, cultural pride, social distinction and consequence. Moreover

11

in ceramics, in all of what are called the applied arts, only a cultural identity, by and large, is likely to survive: indeed, the potter's compulsions, as reflected by his work, will rarely have been apparent beyond his immediate companions, beyond the workshop: we remain very much aware, however, that the Korean dish or Sung bowl was an outcome not only of a tradition to which numerous artists had contributed but of an individual who must have again, in his turn, been subject to the aesthetic compulsion to reflect an ideal of ego structure. The same is often true in the sphere of building. We have arrived at a further reason why the painter may represent all artists: his work usually allows us to discern other syntheses (beyond those of a style and of a culture) that underlie the practice of every kind of art. But whereas architecture does not possess the many facets of painting, it shows us the surfaces that matter most, the 'language': it surrounds us so widely that the art of painting cannot be viewed apart from architectural alternatives, volume and void, light and dark, recession and protrusion, the rough and the smooth. That is not at all to say we would have no sculpture or painting without an example of building, but only that in such case, painting and sculpture would themselves have to find a partial substitute for this absence, just as they tend to do now.

To speak of art is sometimes to estrange ourselves from the artist. He seems today often to be concerned merely with the expression of sensations, maybe sensations to touch and tear and mould material. Nevertheless, whatever he may profess, no artist, old nor modern, with the possible exception of a few child-like or naif painters, achieved his aim without having been fired by already existing works of art, especially by the work of contemporaries. The itch to create in the aesthetic sense is perhaps a thing apart; but it follows that the artist is himself no mean connoisseur of creativeness: he understands art; he could not be much of an artist if he did not, since he is extremely sensitive to what lies together, especially to what is intentionally symbolic. There is no hard-and-fast division between the appreciator and the creator of art. Indeed, whatever his conscious interest or knowledge, I have no doubt that the artist is potentially the most highly-trained appreciator, often confined in range of interest by the preoccupation of his own creative field. This is but to emphasize again in a different manner that art is a cultural activity though the fount be hidden and untutored. Were it otherwise, art would not mirror the whole man, the whole of his capacity. The fire of Van Gogh would have been of small consequence had it not consumed Vincent, the copier of drawings in the *Illustrated London News*, the admirer of Millet, and the near-contemporary of the Impressionists. Some artists today ape an effect that is untutored, but insofar as their work is notable, it will be obvious that they are, as artists, the product of modern museums. Nor do they work now in more isolation than heretofore. On the contrary, the movement, the fraternity, seems more essential: few modern paintings make their utmost point without reinforcement from others.

I sent our gallery director packing, yet he now reappears in the train of artists: we are not interested in his business acumen but in his nose. He and his smart gallery are symbols of the cultural relevance of hard agonies in the studio. Picasso is reported to have said that as a child he could draw like Raphael but that later, as an adult, it had taken him a long time to learn to draw like a child. It seems that the character of our culture has inspired an element of regression: it inspired Picasso's early appreciation of the values of negro sculpture, a very important part of his creativeness. We taste a new humility and a new arrogance, a sophistication and a barbarity in all the people and all the things surrounding us: and I do not use the word 'taste' altogether metaphorically since I would stress the oral component in our attitudes to parts of our environment: as presented by art, I have said,

13

it does not overwhelm us since, as well as in the terms of
envelopment and incorporation, we are shown an aspect of
our environment and 'mental climate' by the painter as an
enclosed object, at arm's length, reflecting what I have called
two basic relationships to objects. They are usually experienced together; in art alone their collusion seems perfected to
the extent that we appear to have the cake and to eat it without a greedy tearing, the object to incorporate and the object
set out and self-contained. Surely the status of this cake is the
one of the 'good' *internal* object, the 'good' breast which, as
Melanie Klein (1957) has repeatedly said, formed and forms
the ego's nucleus, the prototype not only for all our 'good'
objects but, in the unenvious, unspoiling relationship with it,
for happiness.

But it is always a prime error to search only for derivations
that are positive, affirmative. I have not pointed to the fact
that part of the aesthetic compulsion will have a negative
basis in the component of aggression and, perhaps, of organ
deficiency as well as in the threat, perhaps always present, of
incipient confusion. We know of several great painters who
have had ceaseless trouble with their eyes, imaginary or real.
When the trouble has been imaginary we must impute to
them an unconscious sense of guilt, unusually strong, in connection with the greedy, prehensile, and controlling act of
vision as it has appeared to the phantasy in early years. To
observe is partly to control, to be omnipotent: whereas the
exercise of the cruel power continues in the making of art, it
is used also to reconstruct what thereby is dismembered: in
reflecting such combined yet antithetical drives, a work of art
symbolizes the broader integrating processes. The aesthetic
account of integration is an end-in-itself, unlike the stock
syntheses that construct a character type, professional, class,
or national, often valued beyond all other ego projections by
unaesthetic persons. Genius displays a new mending of im-
pulse, of feeling, with such conviction that there issues from

14

it a novel treatment of subject-matter as of form. Cézanne applied a steel-bright knife to pattern and to distance: he introduced love and respect into an extraordinary attack upon his apples and upon the landscapes of his home. His paintings are unified by a play of glinting cuts that both bisect and glorify the contour. It is above all composers who demonstrate easily the varieties, and even the contrariety, implicit in a theme. What twists of combined feelings Mozart contrived within the clear cascade of a chamber work.

Many artists of an opposite temperament to Cézanne's will have availed themselves of his discoveries. Considered psychologically the development of art is no less complicated than the view from any other approach. But I want to stress a factor that has usually been simple, the compulsion to 'get things right' issuing in part from the fear of deformity and of aggressiveness. In the case of naturalistic painting the first test of what 'looks wrong' has been very simple. In drawing a jug how shameful it is that a side should become swollen or should be impoverished, how poignant and sacrilegious the lop-sidedness. Many present-day artists defy this fear and scan the lop-sidedness of our environment: modern art tends to conventionalize ugliness and distortion in the search for comprehensive balances: the vibrant power wanes to correct each enormity without devitalization, since art must reflect as well as affirm: idealism in art has been the face put upon some degree of truth, upon some need of balance amid discord: also the unabashed shape of the deformed jug may have this timeless quality. In the past undeformed shapes have sometimes been balanced in a picture asymmetrically: today we often see deformed shapes balanced squarely.

I have already introduced a negative approach in attributing the development of modern painting partly to the nineteenth-century vulgarization of architecture. Ugliness has strengthened not only confusion but a desire for collapse: in art we will here discern an amalgamation of negative and positive components. A collapsed room displays many more facets than a room intact: after a bombing in the last war, we were able to look at elongated, piled-up displays of what had been exterior, mingled with what had been interior, materializations of the serene Analytic Cubism that Picasso and Braque invented before the first war; and usually, as in some of these paintings, we saw the poignant key provided by some untouched, undamaged object that had miraculously escaped. The thread of life persists, in the case of early Cubist paintings a glass, a pipe, a newspaper, a guitar whose humming now spreads beyond once-sounding walls that have become clean and tactile remains. In such strange surroundings, not altogether unlike the intact yet empty buildings invented by Chirico, the brusque accoutrements of comfort for pavement life, the one of the café, extend a great sense of calm: a simple shape and a simple need emerge from the shattering noise and changing facets of the street. Later work by Picasso is more disturbing, since he has broken off and re-combined parts of the body, often adding more than one view of these part-objects. Disruption of flesh and bone extends to the vitals, but the furor of his genius is such that the sum of misplaced sections does not suggest the parts of a machine: on the contrary, in the translated bodies, as in the rent room, of Guernica, there exist both horror and pathos as well as aesthetic calm: the interior of the body is not represented as a ruined closet but as part of an exterior décor. Similarly, the New York Manager of Picasso's ballet, *Parade*, wore his ribs outside his costume and outside the child's skyscraper attached to his head. In the period known as Synthetic Cubism, Picasso and Braque had joined into whole objects upon tilted table-tops the piled-up abstract bric-à-brac accumulated in Analytic Cubism, to an enfolded effect as fresh as fruit. Strong, jagged pattern, a wrought-iron jointure, the curve of a rib blunt or acute, typify enduring characteristics in the manifold variations of Picasso's art, a giant in our times.

16

The distinctiveness of what we call modern art does not lie in the degree of conventionalization or of distortion or in a total neglect of appearances but in the treating by means of such methods of all experiences as if they were rudimentary; impact takes precedence of the values revealed by the last ripple on the pond. Things are already in bits and must themselves be broken up into absorbable parts. The emphasis upon strong impact is an emphasis not only upon the projection of proprioceptive or interoceptive sensations and images associated with a mere part of the body, but consequently upon the merging or incorporating function that belongs pre-eminently to our relationship with any part-object, in the first place the breast of infanthood: we cannot attribute originally to the infant an awareness of whole or separate objects either visually or imaginatively, only of highly coloured attributes or parts that in their supreme goodness or badness are assimilated with himself. In modern art, then, the wealth of adult experiences is often endowed with this primitive cast that is normally retained at such strength in adult life for some states only, such as sleep. I am here referring to a treatment in the work of art, not entirely to the effect of the work itself, which by definition brings to us also the sense of a whole and self-sufficient object. On the other hand, a unifying simplification of shape (and often a shape's mere exaggeration) to some degree figures in *all* plastic art: it facilitates the clutching impact, the easy identification, characteristic of relationship with a part-object, whereby the world is homogeneous. As well as to observe, Form induces us to partake.

We are not likely to use the word 'imaginative' in connection with modern art. This seems strange if we recall the extraordinary inventions of Picasso, for instance, syntheses of many experiences, many feelings; reflections, very often as well, of numerous cultural *nuances* past and present. Are not his phantasmagorias imaginative by definition? Yet I think

17

that even here we are loath to use the word, though we do so at once in regard to works of the early periods and to his classical reminiscences particularly in the early 1920's, to the horses and giant women by the sea and to echoes of pagan myth in representational drawings, to such a series as the one of the artist with the model. Why do we call these works imaginative whereas we make no immediate call for this word in contemplating the far greater fertility of his more recondite works? I believe the answer to be that they are more recondite in a limited sense only, since they are by no means of a hidden or etiolated manner. While it remains difficult to define the imaginative content, we are strongly aware of a constraint upon us to regard their richness as a stripping, a baring, as a defiance even of the symbolization or image-building attributed to the processes of imagination. Indeed, the word 'imaginative' is no longer in constant employment even beyond the range of professional art. Do we any more say that children are imaginative; or children's drawings? We have come to realize that *all* expressions are symbols of a further meaning. I have asked the question whether a typical child's drawing should be considered imaginative. The answer surely is No: a child's drawing finds the equivalent, without much ado, to a hidden tension in himself: hence the lesson learnt by modern art from child's art. The attempt in modern art to break down the accepted image in favour of primitive entities that it symbolizes, results in the formation of images without resonance from which we withhold the adjective 'imaginative'. In pursuing his spadework on what seems virgin ground, the artist of today sometimes manipulates appearances out of all recognition or refuses altogether to have truck with appearances other than the one of his own painting to which, as by Mondrian, the laws of the cosmos are instantly related: the world comes back with a rush in catalogue explanations, whereas what we value in Mondrian are the sensations of architecture of which we are always in need.

Though the greater part of the art of the world demonstrates varying compromises between two treatments of symbols—we can call them here the classical and modern—I do not think that the rawness of impact rescued by recent generations from primitive art and so prized in our own art today—remember, it means a raw impact of formal relationships no less than of other symbols—is likely to cease in attraction, especially since the art of the world has been assembled in photograph and in museum. But there is this point: the slower art, slower, though as strong, in formal impact, is obsessed with the variety and smooth interpenetration of things that in their sum symbolize an integration and independence of the self and of our objects, maybe at some expense of a blatant (though not an eventual) enveloping power to which I have referred. I submit, therefore, there has not been in the West an art reflective of the entire man as successful as the classical Greek and the Renaissance art at its greatest, which strove to endow symbolic objects with the full value of their own appearances.

All great art commands a strong impact, and all great art records as well the last ripple on the pond. Which aspect will be more needed in the future; will the modern concentration upon impact diminish? I have attempted to isolate the deeper necessity of these emphases: there is obviously unforgettable virtue in both.

Epilogue

My hope is that far from needing a more abstract treatment, what I have written above will have stimulated a modicum of consent to the following very brief summary: it embraces similar propositions I have previously put forward (1955, 1955a, 1958).

19

There is a sense in which we absorb the object of our attention: we speak of absorbing or imbibing knowledge while, for the moment, the rest of the world is excluded. Except for contemplative acts we do not mentally imbibe a thing as an end in itself but as part of a wider activity. Though things and their systems remain outside us, we seem to get to know them by taking them in; for the most part, however, we do not will them to flood through every atom of our being in entering the store of what we call the mind. The work of art, on the other hand, though by definition a complete and enclosed system, strongly suggests to us physical and mental states of envelopment and of being enveloped. These identifications vary from strong manipulation of the object to an absorption of it and a sinking into it; I have used the word 'envelopment' as shorthand. Since art is useless, it exists solely for the contemplative act in which the senses are not the mere vehicles; the appeal is first to them. Two important results follow: as the senses are the feelers by which we apprehend the otherness of outside things, the otherness or object-nature of the work of art is stressed in this act of its contemplation; yet, as I have said, the ruling attention is also engaged by the process of its absorption no less than by the more obvious projecting therein of our feelings. The great work of art is surrounded by silence. It remains palpably 'out there', yet none the less enwraps us; we do not so much absorb as become ourselves absorbed. This is the aspect of the relationship, held in common with mystical experience, that I want to stress, because the no less important and non-mystical attitude to object-otherness in aesthetic appreciation has been better admitted. Aesthetic form immediately communicates, as well as a symbolic image of an integrated ego (Stokes, 1958), the answering image of a reconstituted and independent 'good' object. This object thereupon becomes incorporated with a satisfaction that evokes in turn a more permeating ground for what is felt to be good, and so a symbol for the 'good' breast. The process entails the feeling of 'a pulse in common', of a heightened identification between the appraiser and his object: it is a process that has been accentuated in the so-called conventionalized or conceptual styles of the graphic arts; without ado they impart a generalized image imposed upon what is particular, upon what is mere appearance, transcendent equally of self and of object-nature. Evoking, through the creation of symbolic inducements, the manner of primitive attachment to a part-object (e.g. the breast), art has served ritual, religion, and every cultural aim. In this context, but more particularly outside it, that is to say, in examples which lack the focus of a narrow cultural ideal, we find an employment, as I shall show in the following two essays, for a type of experience that may be called visionary, though coupled (as assuredly it must be in the creation of art) with an insistence upon the independence of a limited, self-sufficient object.

What common analogy can we find for so strong an absorption of ourselves into other things? As a matter of fact such identification is extremely common: an element of it enters into all group attitudes, all states of contemplation and physical engrossment. The most common is surely the state of sleep wherein we discern best the 'oceanic feeling' as Freud called it, a loss of identity that he referred to the infant's satisfaction at the breast with which he is one, a part-object that does not suggest the distinctiveness from its perceiver of a whole object. (There are many methods of confusion with the object, under the stress of predominantly negative feelings, that result in serious loss of ego power. The affirmative quality of aesthetic value I have in mind is bound to be related, largely in a compensatory manner, with these mechanisms of attack and of defence.)

Dr. Lewin's so-called 'dream screen' is 'distinguished from the rest of the dream and defined as the blank background upon which the dream picture appears to be projected. . . . It has a definite meaning in itself' . . . and 'represents the idea of "sleep"; it is the element of the dream that betokens the fulfilment of the cardinal wish to sleep, which Freud considered responsible for all dreaming. Also, it represents the maternal breast, usually flattened out, as the infant might perceive it while falling asleep. It appears to be the equivalent or the continuation, in sleep, of the breast hallucinated in certain pre-dormescent states, occasionally observed in adults' (Lewin, 1948). Whether or not the dream screen is well authenticated, it serves to illustrate the formal value to which I would point in aesthetic experience, usually associated with a subject-matter (the dream itself). In such projections the good breast is of an illimitable character: art is here joined by religious and philosophical yearning for the absolute, so primitive and, some will think, so destructive of good sense in a pretended context of universal truth. The superb place for it is in useless art, harnessed to an equal emphasis upon object-otherness. We must realize at the same time that more generally an oral character in experience is very common; the modes of identification necessary to culture and to cultural behaviour, in part depend upon it.

Thus, in virtue of its form at least, art rehearses favourable relationships free of excessive persecution, greed, and envy. Convention, stylization, the power to generalize, are among the means of furthering the enwrapping component in aesthetic form: where one line does the job of two, in any simplification, we experience the emphasis upon singleness. But at the same time the identical formal qualities, such as pattern, that lend themselves to an envelopment theme, are the means also for creating the object-otherness, independence, and self-containment of the work of art: it 'works' on its own, 'functions' in the way of an organism: this phantasy accompanies the one of our being enveloped, but is connected with another that projects the ego in terms of an integrated figure in which opposite characteristics coalesce.

22

The idea of beauty, I have said elsewhere (Stokes, 1958), projects the integrated ego in the terms of a corporeal figure.

I add this note in regard to Dr. Lewin's description of his dream screen as a flattened breast. One thinks at once of the flattened shapes especially of low relief in much art of the world, particularly Quattrocento low reliefs, often of the Mother and Child; and, more generally, one thinks of the picture plane in painting that is preserved at all costs by modern art: more generally still, one thinks of the little recessions, lines, and protuberances of pilasters, for instance, of the markings on freize or cornice, by which architecture reconstitutes the body. I wrote many years ago: 'Architecture is a solid dream for those who love it. One often wakes from sleeping without any recollection of a dream but conscious of having experienced directions and alternatives and the vague character of a weighty impress in harmony with the non-figurative assertiveness of building. In architectural experience, however, changing surfaces, in-out, smooth-rough, light-dark, up-down, all manner of trustful absorption by space, are activated further than in a dream; full cognizance of space is sign enough of being wide awake. The state of sleep has thus been won for actuality.'

And so, too, I make bold to say, in art altogether.

References

HARTIGAN, GRACE. From the catalogue of *The New American Painting*, an Arts Council exhibition at the Tate Gallery (1959).

KLEIN, MELANIE. *Envy and Gratitude* (London, 1957).

LEWIN, B. D. 'Inferences from the Dream Screen'. *International Journal of Psycho-Analysis*, 1948.

THREE ESSAYS ON THE PAINTING OF OUR TIME

STOKES, A. *Michelangelo: a Study in the Nature of Art* (London, 1955).

STOKES, A. 'Form in Art'. From *New Directions in Psycho-Analysis*, edited by M. Klein, P. Heimann, and R. E. Money-Kyrle (London, 1955a). Reprinted in *Journal of Aesthetics*, Vol. XVIII, No. 2.

STOKES, A. *Greek Culture and the Ego* (London, 1958).

WITTKOWER, R. *Art and Architecture in Italy*, 1600–1750. (Harmondsworth: 1958).

II. SOME CONNECTIONS AND DIFFERENCES
   BETWEEN VISIONARY AND AESTHETIC
   EXPERIENCE

II. Some Connections and Differences between Visionary and Aesthetic Experience

I am not writing on the subject of hallucination as a whole in connection with art. The aspect of adult hallucination with which I am concerned is usually spoken of as mystical or visionary experience.

In a book on colour nearly twenty-five years ago (1937) I tried to divide sharply a characteristic visionary experience of colour from an aesthetic. 'When we shut our eyes', I wrote, 'we see a film of colour that scientists call the visual grey. They distinguish so-called film colour from what they call surface colour on which there is always a perceptible texture or microstructure. . . . 'The visual world'—I should have said the adult visual world—'exists between the film colours of our closed eyes and those of an unclouded sky: as harmonious surfaces in this outer world the artist externalizes and orders the divisions of the ego.' It appears certain, I realize now, that the infant at first sees film colour only. I regarded the experiences of colour that are inseparable from textures to be potentially aesthetic, allowing in the aesthetic effect only a small admixture of the always spongy chromaticism, ill-defined in space, of film colour. I was referring to visionary experience when I wrote: 'The tenuous and rakish mythology of film colour has little or no connection with the general appearance of colour as the attribute of surfaces.'

I think that this judgement was extreme, not only in regard to colour, but in the more general sense of an almost complete separation between visionary and aesthetic experience. Attempting to re-define an aspect of their relation, I hope that I may be discussing to some purpose a quality of their

27

characters. In basing so much on a distinction between film and surface colour, I attempted to indicate the gamut of object-relationship, that is, the distance between the relationship that entails an envelopment with the object and the relationship that preserves intact an independent and separated object. But for many years now I have no longer regarded an enveloping relationship to be foreign to the intention of art: on the contrary, I have thought of it as a fundamental attribute when associated with the opposite relationship to an independent object.

Throughout the book on colour I was very severe, then, on film colour and on any effect allied to it, for instance, in the case of what is burnished or lustrous or sparkling, indeed on all effects most dear to infants and children: severe from the point of view of art, that is. Yet after reading Aldous Huxley's two short books, *The Doors of Perception* (1954) and *Heaven and Hell* (1956), I cannot think that the prejudice was entirely ill-founded. I do not hesitate to draw on these books alone for the few generalizations I want to make about visionary experience, since they are wide-ranging as well as poetic: and Huxley is always excellent about art: moreover there is the advantage that he has not hesitated to relate schizophrenic states with the visionary: the connection exists from the first pages of the first book when he discusses adrenochrome and mescalin, the drug that he took in order to enter what he calls 'Mind-at-large' or, in the second book, 'the mind's antipodes'. He attributes to these experiences (which were not in his case inner visions but glosses upon exterior perception) some awareness of cosmic reality—I think to those that are negative also, undergone particularly in schizophrenia—believing that the superior visionary grasp of essence obtains the attention of consciousness as a result of minimizing what he calls the reducing-valve of the mind, by means of drugs, starvation, flagellation, and other methods whereby the somatic chemistry is altered for the worse from the point of view of coping with ordinary external reality. Mystical illuminations do not tally with what are commonly regarded as normal faculties of mind and body. I believe it is sometimes supposed that extra-sensory perception will be favoured by a similar limitation. Telepathic hallucinations, do they exist, reveal cognizance of actual occurrence beyond ordinary ken in the realm of ordinary fact. On the other hand, the very radiance that bathes the objects of environment in an 'outer' visionary experience is claimed by Huxley and other mystics to partake of an underlying status throughout the cosmos. These experiences at best are thought to oppose the temporality of ordinary existence, point to a final aim, to the reconciliation of opposites, to a merging or loss of self in the impersonal Divine Ground. It is obvious to anyone trained in psycho-analysis that such experiences, no less than the schizophrenic, entail the regression not only to the perceptions, but to concepts, characteristic, in one part, of the primitive ego. I shall have two points in mind when quoting Huxley, the merging with the good breast and a rejection of symbolic meaning. I shall ignore an equally significant aspect, the swift change of the good object into Hell, into the bad.

We encounter, then, a very youthful light; the treasures are mostly of the breast as we are transported into a world blazing with colour. The incidence of visionary experience is usually described as a state of being transported. It has suggested to me the condition of being snatched back partially into infancy but also an image of the infant picked up from the cot and carried to the bed or chair for the feed for which he has pined. Indeed, describing the onset of his mescalin experience, Huxley writes: 'The legs, for example of that chair—how miraculous their tubularity, how supernatural their polished smoothness! I spent several minutes—or was it several centuries?—not merely gazing at those bamboo legs but actually *being* them—or rather being myself in them; or, to be still more accurate (for "I" was not involved in the case,

nor in a certain sense were "they") being my Not-self in the
Not-self which was the chair.' 'There seems to be plenty of
it,' was Huxley's answer to the investigator who asked what
he was feeling about time. But space and distance, he says,
'cease to be of much interest. . . . I saw the books, but was not
at all concerned with their positions in space. What I noticed,
what impressed itself upon my mind was the fact that all of
them glowed with living light.' Whereas, and indeed partly
because, the infant may often be fed in the dark, the breast-
object, when hallucinated, will surely glow with praeternatural light like the solitary candle in a painting by Georges
de la Tour whom Huxley calls a visionary painter. Huxley
refers also to the mysterious force of an illumined figure
against a dark ground and to fireworks and other 'vision-like
effects' that 'have played,' he says, 'a greater part in popular
entertainment than in the fine arts.' He instances pageantry,
theatrical spectacles as well as jewels and flowers.

Visionary colour, he tells us, has the freshness 'of experiences which have never been verbalized.' He has quoted and
condensed Weir Mitchell's account of a peyote-inspired
vision. 'At his entry into that world he saw a host of "star
points" and what looked like "fragments of stained glass."
Then came "delicate floating films of colour." These were
displaced by an "abrupt rush of countless point of white
light", sweeping across the field of vision. Next there were
zigzag lines of very bright colours, which somehow turned
into swelling clouds of still more brilliant hues. Buildings
now made their appearance, and then landscapes. There was
a Gothic tower of elaborate design with worn statues in the
doorways or on stone brackets. "As I gazed, every projecting
angle, cornice and even the faces of the stones at their join-
ings were by degrees covered or hung with clusters of what
seemed to be huge precious stones, but uncut stones, some
being more like masses of transparent fruit. . . . All seemed to
possess an interior light". The Gothic tower gave place to a

mountain, a cliff of inconceivable height, a colossal birdclaw carved in stone and projecting over the abyss, an endless unfurling of coloured draperies, and an efflorescence of more precious stones. Finally there was a view of green and purple waves breaking on a beach "with myriads of lights of the same tint as the waves".'

The Weir Mitchell vision, it will be obvious, projected symbols of primary objects additional to those of the breast or nipple: but where on balance they are beneficent, the *mise-en-scène* at least of such experiences is the nursing situation, if only because of a stress that belongs to my first point, the pleasurable absence of self in a merging with the object, a trusting incorporation both of, and with, an object in a dimension of infinite impersonality. As a matter of fact we never lose the sense of such a feeling since it belongs to a variety of normal somatic experiences at their best. Huxley himself remarks that 'in the nuptial embrace personality is melted down: the individual . . . ceases to be himself and becomes a part of the vast impersonal universe'. 'The more than human personages of visionary experience never "do anything" ', he writes, 'they are content to exist.' He has in mind, of course, what may be called visions of a New Jerusalem rather than horrors of confusion due to attempted control through projective identification, of splitting failure and of persecution, of violent fragmentation into myriad pieces. But even in Huxley's accounts there is a reference beyond the good nursing situation to one of more dubious, if more ancient, comfort. 'Experimental psychologists have found,' Huxley says, 'that, if you confine a man to a "restricted environment", where there is no light, no sound, nothing to smell, and, if you put him in a tepid bath with only one, almost imperceptible thing to touch, the victim will very soon start "seeing things", "hearing things" and having strange bodily sensations.'

He does not ask why, in this case, environment alone

31

should cause visions. We, on the other hand, are interested in these experiences because of the situations and objects they recall through symbols. But the mystic claims that, unlike other images, they symbolize nothing: their essence is their 'is-ness'. 'Charged with is-ness', writes Huxley, 'the percept had swallowed up the concept.' In a further passage he writes: 'Praeternatural light and colour are common to all visionary experiences. And along with light and colour there goes, in every case, a recognition of heightened significance. The self-luminous objects which we see in the mind's antipodes possess a meaning, and this meaning is, in some sort, as intense as their colour. Significance here is identical with being; for, at the mind's antipodes, objects do not stand for anything but themselves. . . . Their meaning consists precisely in this; that they are intensely themselves and, being intensely themselves, are manifestations of the essential givenness, the non-human otherness of the universe.'

Our author himself remarks that for what he calls Mind-at-large, 'the so-called secondary characters of things are primary. Unlike Locke, it evidently feels that colours are more important, better worth attending to than masses, positions and dimensions.' It seems to me he points here to the film colour of which I spoke at the start, a colour-effect distinct from the predominant chromatic usage in painting where colour is linked with surface as a rule, with texture, with objects in space. Film colour, then, in the Huxleyan context, represents the non-symbolic. He writes: 'Colour (for which we can read film colour) turns out to be a kind of touchstone of reality. That which is given is coloured; that which our symbol-creating intellect and fancy put together is uncoloured.' In asking why 'in most dreams the symbols are uncoloured', he writes, 'the answer, I presume, is that, to be effective, symbols do not require to be coloured.' What appears to stand for nothing but itself, to exist as a state of being that prevents any attachment to it of symbolic meaning

32

because, all unknown, it represents the very 'is-ness' of the original object, will be highly coloured, it seems, more highly than the external world of ordinary perception also 'given' of course, but upon which, unlike visionary perceptions, we cannot but consciously (as well as unconsciously) lavish, project, our emotions, causing natural objects in this way to be symbols, as well as things other than the inner states they symbolize.

I find this extraordinary point of view that I have interpreted of the greatest interest, not primarily because of the old distinction I had built upon film colour and surface colour in the context of art. For, on the contrary, this claim that there is a non-symbolic chromatic effect reintroduced to me an aspect of aesthetic endeavour, explaining, to my satisfaction at any rate, a very general compulsion in modern art. I will speak of it in a moment.

Art is the metropolis of symbolic manifestations: we practise therein the rites of symbolism. Consequently, we may practise there as well every mode of perception: witness our interest in children's art and the successful enlargement of uninstructed perceptiveness by modern painters. All art rehearses simultaneously, I insisted in 1951, more than one object-relationship, to a part-object as well as to a whole object. It will symbolize not only the gamut of relationship in a favourable union, but also the two kinds of symbolic content of which I shall speak in a moment, fused more ideally than they are likely to be for long in our living out our lives. Dr. Elliott Jaques claims that the two kinds of symbolic content are mingled in all perception. I will quote from his Congress Paper on Work (1959): 'The perception of an object is determined by the interplay of the requisite content of the percept with two types of symbolic content which have been variously designated; for example, by Hanna Segal as symbols and symbolic equations, and by Ernest Jones as symbols and true symbols. Whatever the terms used for the two types of symbolic content—and many writers, including Marion Milner and Dr. Rycroft, have emphasized the importance of the distinction—the central factor is that stressed by Melanie Klein (and elaborated by Segal), namely, the degree of concreteness of the symbol, and the extent to which it co-exists with the object or engulfs it.' I break off to remind you that whereas we have clearly seen that Huxley's Mind-at-large in general unconsciously symbolizes the breast relationship, we have also discovered that symbolic function altogether is thereby reduced and made narrow: the engulfment of the object is not a subsidiary but *the unique part* of the experience. Huxley quotes Coomaraswamy on the mystical art of the Far East, 'The art where "denotation and connotation cannot be divided. . . . No distinction is felt between what a thing "is" and what it "signifies".' Huxley also quotes what he calls 'the divine tautology, "I am I".'

To come back to Dr. Jaques's paper. 'The degree of concreteness in turn depends upon the intensity and character of the splitting process which underlies the symbol formation. It is consistent with recent developments in Melanie Klein's conception of the paranoid-schizoid position (and indeed with unstated assumptions in her earlier work) to assume that it is when violent splitting with fragmentation of the object and the self is predominant, that concrete rather than plastic symbol formation occurs.'

I had best quote also from the Paper by Hanna Segal (1957) to which Dr. Jaques has referred: 'The early symbols . . . are not felt by the ego to be symbols or substitutes, but to be the original object itself. They are so different from symbols formed later that I think they deserve a name of their own. In my paper of 1950 I suggested the term "equation". This word, however, differentiates them too much from the word "symbol" and I would like to alter it here to "symbolic equation".

'The symbolic equation between the original object and

34

the symbol in the internal and the external world is, I think, the basis of the schizophrenic's concrete thinking where substitutes for the original objects, or parts of the self, can be used quite freely, but, as in the two examples of schizophrenic patients which I quoted, they are hardly different from the original object: they are felt and treated as though they were *identical* with it. This non-differentiation between the thing symbolized and the symbol is part of a disturbance in the relation between the ego and the object. Parts of the ego and internal objects are projected into an object and identified with it. The differentiation between the self and the object is obscured. Then, since a part of the ego is confused with the object, the symbol which is a creation and a function of the ego—becomes, in turn, confused with the object which is symbolized.'

I want to quote as well a few sentences concerning the patients that Dr. Segal mentions: they illustrate so aptly the distinction between the opposing methods of symbolization. 'One', she writes, 'whom I will call A was a schizophrenic in a mental hospital. He was once asked by his doctor why it was that since his illness he had stopped playing the violin. He replied with some violence: "Why? Do you expect me to masturbate in public?"'

'Another patient, B, dreamt one night that he and a young girl were playing a violin duet. He had associations to fiddling, masturbating, etc., from which it emerged clearly that the violin represented his genital and playing the violin represented a masturbation phantasy of a relation with a girl.

'Here then are two patients who apparently use the same symbols in the same situation—a violin representing masturbation. The way in which the symbols function, however, is very different. For A, the violin had become so completely equated with his genital that to touch it in public became impossible. For B, playing the violin in his waking life was an important sublimation. We might say that the main difference between them is that for A the symbolic meaning of the violin was conscious, for B unconscious. I do not think, however, that this was the most important difference between the two patients. In the case of B, the fact that the meaning of the dream became completely conscious had in no way prevented him from using his violin. In A, on the other hand, there were many symbols operating in his unconscious in the same way in which the violin was used on the conscious level.'

In the matters of which I am writing, a degree of implicit symbolic equivalence is, no less than the rest of the deeper symbolism, of course, unconscious. We are encountering, in the aesthetic context also to which I now turn, a symbolic projection of a pull towards symbolic equivalence or concrete thinking that has reached consciousness in terms of a violent reversal whereby an impersonal outer object of an absolute and unrelated character, takes the place of a primary object in its activity of overwhelming symbolic substitutes. Even so, in art at any rate, it is not difficult to discern that there is a degree of concrete thinking at work. I am not referring to a displacement, whereby an idol, for instance, takes the place of a god, just as thumb-sucking can take the place of breast-feeding. As well as being the object it represents, the idol is normally, in part, a true substitute though it be thought to accept sacrifices and to resent ill-usage. I do not doubt that the need for such replacement, together with the earlier need of hallucination, has often inspired creativeness. Professor Gombrich brilliantly evoked this point in his paper about the hobby-horse (1951). Insofar as it denies the element of substitution, concrete thinking goes further. We would not value art as we do unless we found there the counterpart of every paramount symbolic function. Before reading Huxley's two books I had not realized how deeply connected symbolic equations are likely to be with the part-object-envelopment aspect of aesthetic form: but it had been certain that both

36

beliefs and phobias, and the consequent taboo, sometimes associated with image-making, no less than the ban still imposed by some societies on the using of proper names, point to this perennial component in symbolism of symbolic equivalence or concrete thinking.

I have written elsewhere (1958) of pronouncements by Braque: they put me in mind of concrete thinking as he described an aim for the artist that has accompanied a fragmentation in representing people and things, well illustrated by the extraordinary achievements of Cubism. Consider now the words of Kandinsky who was one of the initiators, not only in regard to his own circles of Munich and Russia, but to the very various manifestations that come together, if in no other simple way, under the expression *avant-garde*. Kandinsky conceived that a representation of an object might be an unnecessary middle term between the painter and his picture. 'Modern art', he wrote, 'can be born only when signs become symbols.' 'Point and line,' commented Carola Giedion-Welker, 'are here detached from all exploratory and utilitarian purpose. . . They are advanced to the rank of autonomous, expressive essences, as colours had been earlier.' Kandinsky, a student of Rudolf Steiner and Madame Blavatsky, was exploring a theory of spiritual symbolism, a symbolism for the depths (and doubtless the heights) that has nearly always cropped up in modern movements. It is bound to be a muddled thinking: a demand for a more charged, and often child-like, mode of symbolism alternates with a claim, revealed in the use of such words as 'super-real' or 'ultra-object', that a work of art should 'stand' for nothing, should possess a value entirely without reference outside itself, similar to the manifestations of Huxley's Mind-at-large. We are often put in remembrance of visionary experiences: take the case of the apocalyptic occurrence to Kandinsky himself in 1908. I quote this and other statements from Herbert Read's *Modern Painting* (1959). 'I was returning, immersed in thought,' wrote Kandinsky, 'from my sketching, when on opening the studio door, I was suddenly confronted by a picture of indescribable and incandescent loveliness. Bewildered, I stopped, staring at it. The painting lacked all subject, depicted no identifiable object and was entirely composed of bright colour-patches. Finally I approached closer and only then recognized it for what it really was—my own painting, standing on its side on the easel. . . . One thing became clear to me—that objectiveness, the depiction of objects, needed no place in my paintings, and was indeed harmful to them.'

Since that time in 1908, to whatever school they belong, whatever else they have contained, we have had many paintings whose mere muddled radiance suggests the Huxleyan visionary experience of 'is-ness'. Malevitch announced in 1912 that the reality of art was the sensational effect of colour itself. Already in 1910 the Futurist manifesto had stated 'that motion and light destroy the materiality of bodies': their paintings of what I would call film colour have made it clear. About the same time in Paris, Delaunay declared that 'colour alone is both form and subject'. His were among the first, if not the first, entirely abstract paintings. Herbert Read describes them as 'fragmented rainbows'. I find it significant that abstract art began with such professions. Of course, many later manifestations are of an entirely different character, intent upon geometry, even depth sometimes, and most of all, texture. All the same, the mystical element, in catalogue, in title, in manifesto at least, is not far away, the element of an unstoppable super-reality. Even Expressionist art, it appears, even that insistence on the externalizing of all that may be most rabid in the artist himself in contradistinction to the abstract artist's existentialist announcement that the cosmos *is* the cosmos, has in the end tended the same way: not without reason Action painting in America is sometimes described as abstract

Expressionism. Herbert Read says about Jackson Pollock's later paintings: 'Of symbolism there is no suggestion: on the contrary a desire to destroy the image and its symbolic associations.' Pollock himself spoke of 'concrete pictorial sensations'. His aim was to get inside his own paintings rather than that his paintings should represent what was inside him. Such projective identification, typified in the novel features of what is undoubtedly excellent art, must curtail the extensive creation of symbolism proper. I think it obvious that *avant-garde* painting of the moment has reached the acme in a fully symbolic representation of symbolic equivalence, and I believe we can discover the same tendency in all the *avant-garde* movements, however opposed, even diametrically, to Action painting they otherwise would have been.

I have indicated that the manifestoes of the artists, and of their impresarios, are extremely muddled. How could it be otherwise, inasmuch as art is the succulent *potage* of differing object-relationships and methods of symbolization? There has been a sustained attempt to project through the symbolism of art naked processes of being and the earlier perceptions, an attempt on all sides: artists, we can be sure, have never tried so consciously to reflect untrammelled perception, at the same time to get behind symbols: they have gone to the length of embracing automatism. Some success in regard to the primitive ego or primary process has not eluded them altogether: in a distorted form the mechanism of symbolic equivalence, for instance, has been proclaimed: thus in banishing, or in attempting to banish, any element of illustration, an abstract artist may dispense with an ordinary symbolic focus in favour of impersonal 'essence', by which is meant a primary state of Being. One is told that the painting, or a collection of chance rubbish stuck on a flat surface, is not a picture, but an object, of extra-object import: it symbolizes or illustrates nothing, for it is nothing so secondhand. Even the Cubists of 1910 were talking already of *le tableau-objet*. We will remember Schwitters' collages or Marcel Duchamp's 'ready-mades' and the anti-art distinction of the Dadaists between the indirectness of traditional art and the ruddiness of (irrational) life. Writing of Kandinsky's later paintings Herbert Read uses these words: 'His symbolic language has become wholly concrete or objective, and at the same time transcendental. That is to say, there is no longer, and deliberately so, an organic continuity between the feeling and the symbol which 'stands for' it; there is rather a correspondence, a correlation. In liberating the symbol in this way, Kandinsky created an entirely new form of art. . . To a certain degree sensibility itself became suspect to Kandinsky; at least, he insisted on the distinction that exists between the emotion in the artist to be expressed, which is personal, and the symbolic values of line, point and colour, which are impersonal.'

The blending in art of two kinds of symbolic representation is always subtle. It could be argued that the *trompe l'œil* effect against which all modern art reacted, affirms a drab symbolic equivalence; that much contemporary art, on the other hand, has consciously aimed at symbolizing states of mind through the means of external forms. I think it likely that the romantic insistence upon the symbolic function of art, and the refusal to regard representation merely as such, has facilitated the emergence of far deeper aspects of the compulsion, which itself has grown much greater, towards representing symbolic equivalence, indicated by Cézanne's emphasis (prepared by others) upon the reality of the picture plane at the expense of the naturalistic attempt to deny it for the sake of *trompe l'œil*. The styles of Cubism are, in my opinion, the key study: they will one day be understood to be experiments in new blendings of the symbolic ingredients.

At this point I must interrupt to mitigate two of the misunderstandings that I will seem to have invited. I have often stated a work of art to be a self-inclusive entity that mirrors not only the developed ego's integrative processes but the realization or reconstruction of the independent, self-sufficient, mother, a fruit of the successful outcome from the depressive position. But surely it is easy to grasp that the aim of creating a symbolic self-inclusiveness no less apparent in modern, even abstract, art than in other art, can lend itself to a split-off, ego-object, amalgam that expresses nothing but itself. In many modern styles, independent structure, composition, form, the very skeleton of art, has been freed and isolated, amid the decay of all iconography, from what are felt to be the irrelevant demands of a detailed subject-matter, or even of subject-matter altogether. This dislike of conventional illustrative symbolism has, in my opinion, much bearing on the immediacy of effect, on the 'direct' painting technique, of nearly all our art since the Impressionists and before, an emphasis that is, upon broken surface, upon texture, that co-exists with, and even combines with, a *penchant* for a chromaticism to suggest film colour. Similarly, it is surely easy, as I have indicated already, to understand that there will be communicated under one and the same formal treatment two aspects of primitive ego activity, the suggestion of envelopment (in the nursing situation), together with symbols for the negation of full symbolic projections that accord with a varied, adult world. I have illustrated this connection in visionary experience as offered by Huxley. You will remember that I find in art also an enveloping relationship. And, indeed, no one, I imagine, in writing about architecture and sculpture, will have emphasized more than I have done the gradual light from within, as it seems, of some limestones and marbles especially, not violently but broadly reflected, the inner light as well as surface colour.

I would maintain that the artist has sometimes been most the artist when representing an object seen or visualized at

41

least at arm's length, up to the span of the middle distance, whereby the separate, limited existence of what will be represented is most happily conveyed (and the separateness of the whole matter symbolized). But such is not the *mise-en-scène* of Sung landscape painting, for example, under the influence of Zen Buddhism, not of far-Eastern art generally: it is significant that the Oriental use of the brush has provided an influence on the work of some of the leading American painters today. I return to Huxley: 'Distance lends enchantment to the view', he writes. 'A Sung painting of far away mountains, clouds and torrents is transporting; but so are the close-ups of tropical leaves in the Douanier Rousseau's jungles. When I look at the Sung landscape, I am reminded (or one of my not-I's is reminded) of the crags, the boundless expanses of plain, the luminous skies and seas of the mind's antipodes. . . It is the same with the close-ups. I look at those leaves with their architecture of veins, their stripes and mottlings. I peer into the depths of interlacing greenery, and something in me is reminded of those living patterns, so characteristic of the visionary world, of those endless births and proliferations, of geometrical forms that turn into objects, of things that are for ever being transmuted into other things.' I find here a parallel with my opening remark about film colour, easiest seen either within the closed eyes or else in the furthest sky. Huxley mentions medieval tapestries in connection with the close-up mystical effect, a visionary standpoint alien to the Renaissance inventors of linear perspective, no less alien than would have been the far-Eastern objects of nearby scrutiny 'represented in a state of unrelatedness, against a blank of virgin silk or paper'. And yet. . . It was Uccello, the fanatic of perspective, who painted the magical *Hunt in the Wood* at the Ashmolean. For some time Madonnas continued to be offset by monochrome gold backgrounds. Medieval themes were incorporated by the Renaissance painters: and later, who would suggest that the impersonal observation, the studious calm communicated by Vermeer's interiors is not transfiguring? All masterpieces are transfiguring if we mean by this last word that we are taken up into them. They differ in their effect from visionary objects in that they also symbolize an unchanging object-outwardness or sufficiency and an adult integration of the ego. If such are the terms used, art will be defined as a symbolic reduction of experience whereby primitive ego mechanisms, that appear also in visionary experience, reinforce adult perceptions and the adult need to reconstruct a whole and self-sufficient object; an activity, then, whereby an element of symbolic equivalence reinforces true symbolism. I believe all art, when observed from the side of its form, even anti-humanist art, projects an image of the body and the integrated mind, symbolizes a sensuous object-character distinct from ourselves and from the kaleidoscopic brightness it may include, the unitary undertone, of visionary envelopment. Our own stability walks hand in hand with the stability of objects. When culture is attuned to actual or potential traumatic experience, famine, earthquake, pestilence, to privation and persecution or to cultural chaos, art increases its abstraction. I think the tendency can be sometimes illustrated over long periods (Abell, 1957). If this is so, then an enlargement of traumatic experience that threatens to overwhelm the ego, wherein the ego's counter-attack and the experience itself are somewhat confused, will entail for art an increase of the symbolic use of symbolic equivalence: direct representations, either of the traumatic condition or of its cause, will yield to a symbol embracing both of them with an air of impersonality and even of 'is-ness'. In any case, in spite of ego-integration, we all of us, as ever, contain extremely good and extremely bad objects that do not come together nor limit each other: we still employ distorting mechanisms of defence that make for some confusion between ego and objects. While art, all art, in whatever degree,

43

separates those terms, it symbolizes primitive states as well: the appeal of form is, in part, oral, encompassing, enveloping.

For epilogue, I ask you to contemplate an experience—I think the apprehension resulting from it should be called aesthetic—of the greatest importance to Ruskin as he himself realized, an experience not unconnected, I feel, with a basket of wild, nipple-like strawberries that I would liken to the 'transparent fruit' of Weir Mitchell's vision.

During the past year the young Ruskin had spat blood and was removed from his college at Oxford. In a state of depression he went abroad once more with his parents, looking for health. He writes in his autobiography, *Praeterita*, that when they got to Fontainebleau: 'I lay feverishly wakeful through the night, and I was so heavy and ill in the morning that I could not safely travel, and fancied some bad sickness was coming on. However, towards twelve o'clock the inn people brought me a little basket of wild strawberries; and they refreshed me, and I put my sketch-book in pocket and tottered out, though still in an extremely languid and woebegone condition; and getting into a cart-road among some young trees, where there was nothing to see but the blue sky through the branches, lay down on the bank by the roadside to see if I could sleep. But I couldn't, and the branches against the blue sky began to interest me, motionless as the branches of a tree of Jesse on a painted window.

'Feeling gradually somewhat livelier, and that I wasn't going to die this time, and be buried in the sand, though I couldn't for the present walk any further, I took out my book, and began to draw a little aspen tree, on the other side of the cart-road, carefully.

'How I managed to get into that utterly dull cart-road, when there were sandstone rocks to be sought for, the Fates, as I have so often to observe, only know. . . And today, I

44

missed rocks, palace, and fountain all alike, and found myself lying on the bank of a cart-road in the sand, with no
prospect whatever but that small aspen tree against the
blue sky.

'Languidly, but not idly, I began to draw it; and as I drew,
the languor passed away: the beautiful lines insisted on being
traced—without weariness. More and more beautiful they
became, as each rose out of the rest, and took its place in the
air. With wonder increasing every instant, I saw that they
"composed" themselves by finer laws than any known of
men. At last, the tree was there, and everything that I had
thought before about trees, nowhere. . . This was indeed an
end to all former thoughts with me, an insight into a new
sylvan world.

'Not sylvan only. The woods, which I had only looked on
as wilderness, fulfilled I then saw, in their beauty, the same
laws which guided the clouds, divided the light, and balanced
the wave. "He hath made everything beautiful, in his time",
became for me thenceforward the interpretation of the bond
between the human mind and all visible things; and I re-
turned along the wood-road feeling that it had led me far;
—further than ever fancy had reached, or theodolite
measured.'

It was a visionary and also an aesthetic experience: it
marked the waning of a period of hypochondria and of
psychosomatic illness: in the forms of an exterior perception
Ruskin regained the measure of a good incorporated object
and of potency feeling, focused by the integrated body of
the aspen tree. The occasion was nearest prepared by the
manic impact upon him of the basket of strawberries: we
cannot doubt it. Nearly thirty years later, two years before
his first entire mental breakdown, Ruskin was recording
dreams. On the night of November 11–12th, 1869, he
dreamed of what he calls 'a friend of mine' running a race,
who asked for a basket of strawberries from a girl walking

in front. 'So I ran and caught her, and she had four little baskets of strawberries, all stuck together and I couldn't choose which basket to take.' Later in the dream he has the same difficulty of choice about cakes in a baker's shop. Two nights after he dreamed again about cakes, some of which were too rich and others too poor: finally a customs man in France drank so much of his, Ruskin's, magnificent old brandy, that Ruskin told him that since he had already had more than half the bottle he might as well have the lot: 'and I came away very angry: and awoke.'

Poor Ruskin's good objects, at that time, particularly the wild strawberries of the child, Rose la Touche, were the centre of unceasing conflict. Art might have saved him—it did so repeatedly—but as a tortured unappeased visionary, entranced by the utterly good, imprisoned without warning by an unutterable bad, he was finally doomed: so it seems at first sight. The last words of the last entry in his diary, the only one for 1889, before the attack of mania that incapacitated him for work during the remaining ten and a half years of his life, most unusually reports the remark of a child he calls Baby, on waking in the mother's room: 'do you know, mother, looking at that beautiful picture of these melons is quite a feast to me' (Evans, 1959). As I have said, this is the last entry, before confusion descended, of diaries Ruskin had written during some fifty years.

It appears a fair conclusion for the whole of this essay to affirm, or maybe to re-affirm, that the manic defence, insofar as it resumes a process either of splitting or of confounding, in fact flirts with schizoid methods. Such is the bridge, it appears, between the predominantly manic-depressive temperament of the artist and his visionary bent, his symbolic projection of concrete thinking.

46

References

ABELL, W. *The Collective Dream in Art* (Cambridge, Mass., 1957).

ETTLINGER, L. D. *Kandinsky: 'At Rest'* (Oxford, 1961).

EVANS, J, & WHITEHOUSE, J. H. *The Diaries of John Ruskin*, Vol. I, 1835–47, Vol. II, 1848–73, Vol. III, 1874–89 (Oxford, 1956, 1957, 1959).

GOMBRICH, E. H. 'Meditations on a Hobby Horse or the Roots of Artistic Form' from *Aspects of Form* edited by L. L. Whyte (London, 1951).

HUXLEY, A. *The Doors of Perception* (London, 1954).

HUXLEY, A. *Heaven and Hell* (London, 1956).

JAQUES, E. 'Disturbances in the Capacity to Work' *International Journal of Psycho-Analysis* (1960).

READ, H. *The Concise History of Modern Painting* (London, 1959).

SEGAL, H. 'Notes on Symbol Formation' *International Journal of Psycho-Analysis* (1957).

STOKES, A. *Colour and Form* (London, 1937 and 1946).

STOKES, A. 'Form in Art', from *New Directions in Psycho-Analysis* edited by M. Klein, P. Heimann, and R. E. Money-Kyrle (London, 1955).

STOKES, A. *Greek Culture and the Ego* (London, 1958).

III. IS-NESS AND AVANT-GARDE

III. Is-ness and Avant-garde

'I habituated myself,' wrote Rimbaud, 'to simple hallucination: I would see quite honestly a mosque instead of a factory . . . I ended by finding sacred the disorder of my intelligence' (quoted by Wilson, 1931). Any indication of the extremely good and bad in disorderly alternation, of disconnection and of compulsive equivalence, was sacred. At nineteen Rimbaud turned his back on discoveries of the deeper self through art. Not so Alfred Jarry (1873–1907) whose influence upon Apollinaire and Picasso was considerable as well as later upon the Surrealists. He tried to live, says Roger Shattuck, 'in foolish competition with his own work.' He 'refused the contradictions of which he was so keenly aware and asserted the equivalence of all things'. 'The time,' adds Shattuck of the 1900's, 'acknowledged the vitality of certain areas conventionally called evil and lunatic' (Shattuck, 1959). (Almost a hundred years earlier Géricault had painted the portraits of psychotics not as straight grotesques but as complicated human beings.) The element of what we now call anti-art has arisen from an exaggeration of a single aesthetic component, in the determination, as well as from the compulsion, to regress, to embrace, whatever appears more primary, to disconnect in order to bring extraneous things together so that they sprawl at all angles. These manifestations, however, stress a yearning for simultaneity, singleness, and equivalence, in due proportion proper to aesthetic experience, being an aspect of the romantic merging or identification with the object upon which the art of the last 150 years has tended to insist. Owing

51

to this stress, the concomitant search in art for 'the inner man' has often taken a most regressive form. But the 'primitive' has then become sacred only when romantically shorn of its huge components, guilt and anxiety; in fact, there has been the attempt to deny a developed superego in favour of a freedom that must be negatively defined. Jarry, it seems, felt himself free not to be himself, free to enjoy a deliquescence of his ego in favour of a histrionic personage whose performance was re-created each moment like a work of art.

The birth of the *avant-garde* was a long, prodigious labour: scores of years of research are needed for the critical reconstruction. As always, the nature of art is involved. To the indications already attempted, I add a few from preceding historical phases.

I think everyone concurs about the principal point of departure, the Romantic movement, partly prepared in the eighteenth century and before. The French Revolution was, of course, the epoch-making outer event: the stress upon 'isness' in contemporary art is still, it seems to me, a modern version of a romantic reaching for the moon. Not only did the Romantic poet vindicate 'the rights of the individual against the claims of society as a whole', but, 'with his turbid or opalescent language, his sympathies and passions which cause him to seem to merge with his surroundings, he is the prophet of a new insight into nature' (Wilson, 1931): particularly human nature in the manifold 'spiritual' relationships with objects which at the same time were seen to symbolize inner states. Thus, portrayal was known to be self-exploration in a manner more intrusive than heretofore. At the end of the nineteenth century the Symbolists were probing intimations of meaning that escaped from descriptiveness, while their opponents, the Naturalists, likewise infused the interstices of actuality with temperament. In all art of worth a new emphasis lay on the character and act of the performer behind the work, because art seemed to be creating culture rather than culture art: the individual's, the artist's achievement with himself, could appear to be more stable than society's achievement; or so the artist felt. Aesthetic qualities, formal qualities, were nearer to becoming the ego-ideal which, according to my diagnosis, they in fact should be, since they have for their subject-matter the ego's integrative processes. An isolating of the aesthetic content had begun. A subject and its treatment in our own day may be comfortably, or uncomfortably and vulgarly, opposed, whereas in the past a theme might be tragic, petty, or bestial, but its treatment, that is to say, an evident selection in the presentation of incident, had to convey a sense of fitness to which formal qualities will have lent themselves. We now often rely on formal qualities alone for the communication of calm and integration, without any of the helps of conventional appropriateness from the subject. Our artists, then, may forego the air of generality imposed upon the prosaic, or of poetry, the reference to the characteristic, needed hitherto to join with qualities more specifically formal in epitomizing, in symbolizing, the impersonal image of corporeal wholeness and psychical integration. For this reason, not only the selection of subject-matter, but subject-matter itself, has appeared to be of less importance in the making of art; whereas in the past the connection of form and subject-matter through the medium of generalization or convention has always been the very hinge that connected values purely aesthetic and the cultural values that all art serves.

Today the cultural ideal is at best the value of aesthetic process stripped of the elaboration that precise cultural ideals in the past have inspired. We represent, so far as we represent, a non-ideal conception of our surroundings or situation, confused yet forceful. A harsh and often vulgar disclaimer may intervene betwixt an anti-ideal conception and the beauty of its treatment. Beauty, of course, abject beauty, still abounds, *calme, luxe et volupté*, even in contemporary art. It is true,

53

though, in general to say that 'uplift' or sublimity gained from art, a reconciliation with cultural endeavour, with humanitarian judgement, the titillation of the superego, have been transformed into ego-ideal constructions, *tout court*, into manifestations of an aesthetic process through which an individual, as has the artist, may 'find himself'; into naked models of each kind of striving encounter with our objects. We have in common a complete lack of the iconographic symbols that once enabled the arts to build symbolic structures of an evident cultural ramification. Indeed the wish to cut out all the 'nonsense', to symbolize by art 'the inner man' alone, may be said to have reinforced the ambition to possess by means of art an object rather than the symbol for it, to have stimulated, then, the constant desire for the homogeneous state I have called 'is-ness', and so, an impatience with any symbol for it and therefore, in truth, with art itself, the very means by which it may be communicated through the symbolic representation of symbolic equivalence. Hence the vulgar strain in anti-art movements.

A further paradox follows. I have mentioned that in speaking of modern art we do not call much on the word 'imagination'. Indeed, we think of visions and hallucinations as forced upon the recipient, squeezed in, as it were, between his eye-lids by an outside agency or from the depths of his mind, rather than as an active construction of the image-making faculty. This means that for what we regard to be specifically imaginative we retain the sense of a projection whose contents are better related the further they are transposed into a fictitious context, whereas to visionary experience we attribute no intellectual artifice. Baudelaire based his criticism of pictorial Realism (Courbet) a hundred years ago on a not entirely dissimilar conception of the imaginative role. Nevertheless, Baudelaire, likewise the Symbolists who were his heirs, emphasized a visionary grasp of the Real in aesthetic comprehension; a grasp that enclosed an interchange of effects between the different arts themselves. One need have no such theory in order to say, as I have said, that a unitary or visionary quality with which we may identify ourselves has entered into the creation of all art: the Old Masters' building up of monumental treatment to form a varied experience, very often causes the visionary kernel to be the more magical, an illumination for much circumstance whereby also the spectator's adult ego is notably served and flattered.

With whom shall we contrast Tintoretto? The 'Douanier Rousseau's entire career was devoted to creating the universe of a grown-up child. . . . He incarnates his universe by painting it exhaustively and palpably close'. There is 'a single mysterious lighting from all sides, shadowless, without high lights, without any power to dissolve colour' (Shattuck, 1959). Or 'he imagines a strongly lighted distance against which he silhouettes darker forms of tree and foliage. . . . Usually two small figures focus the eye on the foreground. This same "dream picture" haunted him from the days of *Carnival Evening* to the last jungle picture he painted' (quoted in Shattuck, 1959).

Such sentences will call to mind the visionary experiences discussed in the last essay. Picasso's banquet for Henri Rousseau in 1908 was undoubtedly a most significant occasion in the history of the *avant-garde*. Rousseau's pictorial dreams, elaborated in quiet suburbs during an age of some security, crystallize the contribution to *avant-garde* art of the naïve, the bright, and particularly of an unswerving mildness or matter-of-factness in regard to them. It could be argued that this matter-of-factness, often employed for the presentation of even imperfectly induced visions, constitutes one of the characteristics of modern art, separating it from Delacroix's vast visionary exploits, from the last great artist to be taken up with the forging of grandeur. Any masterpiece of the imagination contrasts with a truly child-like matter-of-factness.

E   55

The bridge has long been built between what is considered to be child-like and what is considered to be primitive. Champfleury, the champion of Courbet in the 1850s, is quoted by Professor Schapiro as having written: 'The idol cut in the trunk of a tree by savages, is nearer to Michelangelo's Moses than most of the statues in the annual salons', because of a vividness in common, because of 'signs of a conception' paramount in children's drawings as Rodolphe Töpffer, the Swiss educationalist, remarked in a book of 1848 (Schapiro, 1941). Some interest, then, even in the middle of the nineteenth century, some respect, had begun to be paid to the art of the child and of the savage. Professor Schapiro points out that Courbet was influenced by naïve popular prints. We can easily see that Courbet's art, so revolutionary in that he was absorbed by aesthetic contemplation of his ordinary experience at the expense of the selectiveness or appropriateness to art which was still demanded, has a mindless, visionary quality: it causes the easy justice in his perception of tone, his extraordinary naturalism, to possess an air, unique for the time, of lack of contrivance. Courbet held some devices in contempt: he was accused of being clumsy, childish, mindless, of discovering 'everything in life and nature equally interesting', to quote a criticism in 1860 of the realistic novel (Boas, 1938). A contemporary critic of his *Young Woman on the Banks of the Seine* remarked that their significance was no greater than that 'of two good white cows with russet markings' (quoted in Goldman, 1959). The very accuracy in the wide sweeps of Courbet's observation, allied to a visionary mildness extended equally to all parts of a painting, seemed to make his subject-matter of neutral and even of secondary importance. His matter-of-fact attitude to the nude was felt to be particularly unfeeling. Courbet, wrote Zola, 'had the rugged desire to clasp true life in his arms, he wanted to paint in a meat and potatoes way' (quoted in Goldman, 1959). In so doing he did not envisage as a rule,

56

though he was reviled for left-wing sympathies, a parable of peasant life or of poverty, unlike Millet whose more revolutionary social consciousness cast his art into a traditional symbolic mould. Few of Courbet's works 'possess any humanitarian fervour' (Goldman, 1959). It is easy to understand that the broad back of a 'message' serves in art of however recent a date, a similar rôle to the conscious cultural expressions undertaken by the art of the past. That is why Pissarro considered the transcendental symbolism, re-introduced in a modern idiom by Gauguin and Bernard, to be vulgar and reactionary.

The general reflection in all art, even modern art, of culture is an entirely different case of symbolism. To us it becomes obvious, very obvious, that the Impressionists painted, symbolized by their paintings, 'the good life of the resurgent middle-class', particularly those people as they took their Sunday pleasures. Among artists at work at that time, more than others the Impressionists were the spokesmen of a positive aspect in their age, not merely of a minor spirit in that age. Yet Philippe Burty, one of the earliest admirers of Impressionist painting, justly wrote: 'Man is really an object of interest by virtue of his existence as a fact, the most interesting of all objects, perhaps, but not essentially different from trees, clothes, or the sky.' Thoré, a very perceptive critic, wrote: 'Manet's . . . real vice is a sort of pantheism which values a head no more than a slipper; which sometimes even grants a greater importance to a bouquet of flowers than to the face of a woman' (quoted in Sloane, 1951). The word 'pantheism' is of interest to us in view of the vision we had in the last essay of a transporting and unitary chromatic world. As in the case of Courbet, Realism could be equated by hostile critics with indifference, indifference not only to the object represented but to an acceptable balance of contrasts. An abstractedness, away from the particular object, is not far in the future.

We are at a sufficient distance occasionally to class the great antagonists, Delacroix and Ingres, together (though Baudelaire in 1855 classed Ingres and Courbet) since each was a champion of a narrow cause that piled the fires or cooled the metal of the past. The alternatives of dying traditions were giving less and less scope to the more evident compulsive or personal approach with which they were infused by those few artists who could still successfully improve upon them with stern exaggeration. The difficulty was greatest for the ordinary 'history' painters. 'The nobility of the second Empire, like that of the first, was largely improvised' (Boas, 1938). This once dominant theme ('history' painting) had long been dethroned, at any rate in Holland. Already in the eighteenth century other qualities in art than nobility had been more esteemed (Schapiro, 1954). As well as the Dutch, supporters of Courbet might invoke Caravaggio, Velasquez, Ribera, Chardin, the Le Nain, and Goya. The ordering of the world by art, we have seen, was now to be attributed to the act of the artist independently of any nobility afforded by selectiveness in subject-matter. The Old Masters were persuasive celebrants: modern art invites the communicant, not to share an established ritual, but to contemplate a personal process. It is perhaps more companionable, no more so than the sublime work of Rembrandt who sent his inner being to inhabit the twilight of the Grand Manner. But much of our painting has at least made it clearer that the artist's work must bear witness to the immediacy of outer objects by which we live, as well as to a system of unified parts in the self. Also, we have seen, there has entered some impatience with symbolic function in favour of original, unrelated states.

These are matters that do not figure specifically in artists' manifestoes. It would even be a considerable mistake to suppose that either Courbet or Manet repudiated as such the wider symbolic functions of art. Courbet called his *Burial at Ornans* 'un tableau historique' and his *L'Atelier* 'Allégorie

Réelle', in competition with the old symbolic style. Manet's *Christ and Angels* was exhibited in the Salon of 1864; his *Execution of the Emperor Maximilian* was exactly a 'history' painting. What he felt about the incident will have appeared cool, translated into confronting patches of light and dark material at the expense of supporting anecdotal references. The implications—they would seem entirely unwitting—of any such treatment are more clearly understood in the case of Cézanne. His boyhood friend, Zola, was Manet's most influential supporter. The doctrine of art for art's sake was given in Zola's version by his famous phrase: 'A work of art is a corner of creation seen through a temperament' (quoted in Sloane, 1951). Courbet, he felt, no less than Manet, had set down without preconception his own impressions: the artist was taking a larger hand, were he Realist or Symbolist, in deciding on the very nature of *his* world: otherwise Zola's phrase would be equally applicable to the work of Raphael. More stability or reassurance, it was beginning to be felt, could be enjoyed in contemplating the artist's personal and non-rhetorical emotion than from his protestations however imaginative. Indeed, the very process of aesthetic contriving can be in evidence, at the same time as the painting or composition that results from it: what once would have been judged sketches were now paintings. We see today that the pictorial impact of Cézanne's monumental recreation of objects, in part depends on the concomitant inner adaptation that his recreated objects stabilize. 'The qualities of the represented things', writes Meyer Schapiro in his book about Cézanne (1952), 'simple as they appear, are effected by means which make us conscious of the artist's sensations and meditative processes of work; the well-defined, closed objects are built up by a play of open, continuous and discontinuous, touches of colour. The coming into being of these objects through Cézanne's perceptions and constructive operations is more compelling to us than their meanings or relation to our desires, and evokes in us a deeper attention to the substance of the painting.' That is to say, to speak in the jargon I have used, we are very aware in his painting of a noble ego-integrative activity both in itself and in relation to objects, a prime subject-matter as I have repeatedly said, of the formal element in every art.

Professor Schapiro continues: 'The marvel of Cézanne's classicism is that he is able to make his sensing, probing, doubting, finding activity a visible part of the painting and to endow this intimate, personal aspect with the same qualities of noble order as the world he has imaged. He externalizes his sensations without strong bias or self-assertion. The sensory element is equally vivid throughout and each stroke carries something of the freshness of a new sensation of nature. The subjective in his art is therefore no isolated capricious thing, but a manifestation of the same purity as the beautiful earth, mountains, fruit, and human forms he represents.'

'If I think, everything is lost,' wrote Cézanne. 'What was lost', Lawrence Gowing commented, 'was the pure character of sensation: his whole preoccupation was with perception, and not with receiving only—his attitude was far from the passivity of the pure Impressionist—but with gathering and grasping. Every touch on his canvas adds a new segment to a composite definition, uninfluenced by any that went before. The only consistency is the consistency of sensation, the kinship of one observation with another, progressively evaluated by the meditative eye. Cézanne's method, as he once said, was "hatred of the imaginative", and we can feel that the hatred extended to all that was implied in the derived, fictitious contour of the early works. A picture now showed not only form but the history of its perception: the process of representation was made visible. Painting had in fact become the positive, appreciable action which Cézanne sought, an act of self-possession fit to measure against the world. The artist is not

60

inferior to nature; as he said, "He is parallel with it, unless he deliberately intervenes" ' (Gowing, 1954).

The reader may find in Cézanne's quoted remarks echoes of a visionary approach as I have described it. Far more significant was the utter devotion to Form's perennial symbolic content in regard to ego integration, the process, it seems to me, that Schapiro and Gowing so ably recount in different ways. The freeing of this content, I would suggest, is the most valuable aspect of the art of our time. I have needed to stress also, however, the concurrent enlargement of symbolic representations of symbolic equivalence or concrete thinking. In this respect there is not, of course, a straight line of development stretching from Courbet, say, to the absurdities of Dada: at every point until this last, various syntheses attempt to weld bareness, immediacy, obscurity even, with the activities of the developed ego, and *vice versa*. Thus Gauguin, while he re-introduced a cult of transcendental symbolism, forcing upon his subject-matter generalized meanings other than the aesthetic, employed flat areas of brilliant hue in his paintings, which suggest the non-symbolic 'is-ness' of film colour. 'Beyond the head,' wrote Van Gogh to his brother about a portrait he was painting at Arles, 'instead of painting the banal wall of the mean room, I paint infinity, I make a plain background of the richest, intensest blue that I can contrive, and by this simple combination of the bright head against the rich blue background, I get a mysterious effect, like a star in the depth of the azure sky' (quoted in Schapiro, 1951).

I think it permissible to identify in one of its aspects the 'over-allness', characteristic of so much modern painting, with the visionary stamp of 'is-ness'. This character was stabilized by the immense achievement of Seurat, though he was in every way the antithesis of a mindless painter. There has never been an artist who declared more vehemently a close connection between art and science, who held with greater fervour that everything in a painting should have resulted from the artist's thoughtful participation. No less than Holbein's should Seurat's work be thought the antithesis of Action Painting. Even the smallest of his divisionist paintings are monumental, accumulated, in prolonging a scene or events in a scene. Yet, while he gives painstaking self-inclusiveness to the objects he represents, the striking immediacy of the picture plane insists upon identity of all its parts, an emphasis not so much upon unity as upon oneness.

In discussing the course of modern art it is usual to give more attention than I have done to increasing uses of abstraction. I do not believe that the isolating, which has undoubtedly occurred, of aesthetic formal values, necessarily entails even partial rejection of contingent subject-matter or of its appearances. When I read that the Cubist painter Juan Gris wrote: 'It is not picture X that manages to correspond with my subject, but subject X that manages to correspond with my picture' (quoted in Kahnweiler, 1947); I am reminded that Flaubert, sometimes hailed as the greatest exponent of Realism, could protest that art was more real to him than the events in life. No: one difficulty about subject-matter, however dim or distorted its use, lies with a disturbance that particularization of object-character may bring to bear upon the experience of 'is-ness', upon an experience as well of many things that are yet felt totally to merge into one note.

But some of our most admired younger painters today, whose pictures to the casual glance appear to be total abstractions, repudiate this impression as entirely false. Such an artist claims that he cannot work without the conviction that his painting will be the equivalent, the strongly vibrating equivalent, though in no sense the mere representation, of an outer experience. Both experiences are, as it were, equal in authenticity, the secret experience that inspires the painting and the painting intended to inspire the beholder. The painting is not the symbol of the first experience nor its record:

62

there is no uncertainty on this point: the word used is 'correspondence': the painting corresponds with the experience. This attitude appears to be a form of compromise imposed upon a predominantly 'is-ness' aim.

Few as they are in proportion to the data to be had on every side, I have given sufficient examples, and explained enough, the symbolic projection of symbolic equivalence in modern painting, a quality that, together with the formal values entailed in reconstructing the self and the object, have been cut clear by this art which so nakedly explores 'the inner man' amid cultures that are otherwise disrupted.

I have been using the term 'form' in an unavoidably loose way, to cover the many processes by which the work of art unifies factors for the pleasure of the senses and the mind; to denote, for instance, the symbolic reconciliation of three dimensions with the two of the picture plane, or of contrasted rhythms and movements, or of shapes that are likely to achieve balance in a way that depends upon other modes of reconciliation; to denote the absorption of accents into a whole, the stimulation of bodily as well as intellectual awareness to feel this wholeness; more generally, to denote the bringing together of different kinds and different levels of significance into a cluster: a conception of wholeness underlies every effect. Throughout these essays I have attributed to the aesthetic awareness of wholeness two opposite yet combined *nuances*, the one an experience of singleness or envelopment, the other a recognition of a reconstructed and independent object. The envelopment pull in graphic art, where it notably serves the 'is-ness' asseveration, the confusing of the symbol as of subject with object, I would now designate, perhaps surprisingly, the Pygmalion theme, in honour of the most vulgar of all parables about the nature of graphic art. The life-like statue comes in fact to life; the statue *is* the Woman; *trompe l'oeil*, symbolic equivalence, can do no more.

63

On the other hand, naturalistic art, though it incorporates, as does all graphic art, the Pygmalion theme, may honour better than conceptual or iconic styles an artifact's independence and self-sufficiency, as the result of a more 'objective' mode in observing the outer world, a mode wherein a place can be found in art for recording what is incidental. We have seen that, unlike mystical experience, aesthetic experience depends upon a fair modicum of a less appropriating appreciation of the outer world, in combination with the other attitude.

Having thus treated (in the context of graphic art) of two opposing *nuances* belonging to the effect gained from art, I must briefly restore each to the other. The secret of their combination must lie with the very structure of symbol-formation. According to Freud, the primary mental processes (observable in the analysis of dreams), mechanisms such as those of condensation, projection, and displacement create, at this primitive level, equivalences between meanings that form a cluster of significance in which no one meaning appears to have precedence of another, as does an object have precedence of its symbols for normal and developed consciousness. A grouping of significance, to some extent comparable, figures in art; the very roundness of the aesthetic cluster, even the symbolic reconstruction itself of whole and self-sufficient objects, the aesthetic entity separate from its creator, contains, from the process of its manufacture, more than a trace of the primitive habit of mind, which, while providing the genetic basis of symbol-formation, can be so subject to the paranoid-schizoid stress as to inhibit a continuing development therefrom of true symbolism: in art an outcome may be a symbolic projection of symbolic equivalence or concrete thinking whose poetry becomes disproportionate to an aesthetic end.

We have seen that important aspects of the nature of graphic art, pre-eminently this one, have been abstracted a little from the past and put on view in semi-isolation by our heroes of the *avant-garde*.

References

BOAS, G. (Ed.) *Courbet and the Naturalist Movement* (Baltimore, 1938).

GOLDMAN, B. 'Realist Iconography: Intent and Criticism.' *Journal of Aesthetics*, Vol. XVIII (Baltimore, 1959).

GOWING, L. Catalogue to Arts Council Cézanne Exhibition (London, 1954).

KAHNWEILER, D. H. *Juan Gris, His Life and Work*. Trans. D. Cooper (New York, 1947).

SCHAPIRO, M. Review of Sloane (1951) in *Art Bulletin*, June, 1954.

SCHAPIRO, M. 'Courbet and Popular Imagery.' *Courtauld-Warburg Journal*, Vol. IV, (London), 1941.

SCHAPIRO, M. *Vincent Van Gogh* (London, 1951).

SCHAPIRO, M. *Paul Cézanne* (New York, 1952).

SHATTUCK, R. *The Banquet Years* (London, 1959).

SLOANE, J. *French Painting between the Past and Present: Artists, Critics, and Traditions*, 1848–70 (Princeton, 1951).

WILSON, E. *Axel's Castle* (New York, 1931).

For Product Safety Concerns and Information please contact our EU
representative GPSR@taylorandfrancis.com
Taylor & Francis Verlag GmbH, Kaufingerstraße 24, 80331 München, Germany